STOMACH ULCER DIET COOKBOOK FOR SENIORS

Healthy anti-inflammatory recipes to naturally manage and support digestive system

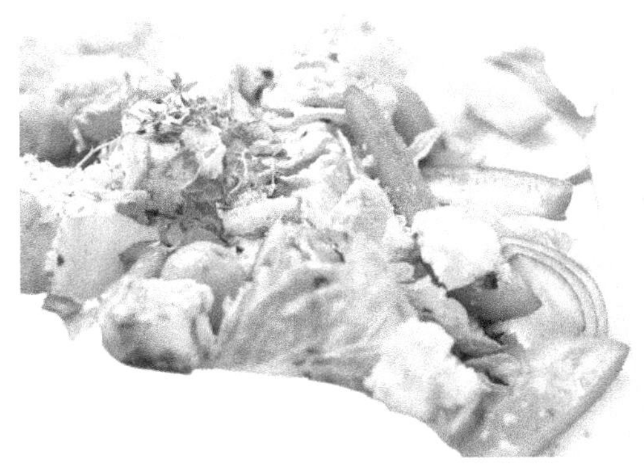

Dr. Malvin Harison

TABLE OF CONTENT

INTRODUCTION

Understanding Stomach Ulcers in Seniors

Gastric ulcers, commonly referred to as stomach ulcers, are lesions that form on the inner lining of the stomach. In seniors, these ulcers can be a common health concern, often influenced by a combination of factors such as age, lifestyle, and pre-existing health conditions.

As the body ages, the stomach lining may become more susceptible to damage, and seniors may experience a higher incidence of stomach ulcers compared to younger individuals. Understanding the intricacies of stomach ulcers in the context of aging is crucial for effective management and prevention.

This section delves into the definition, causes, and prevalence of stomach ulcers among seniors, offering a comprehensive overview to establish a foundational understanding.

Importance of a Specialized Diet

A crucial aspect of managing stomach ulcers in seniors revolves around adopting a specialized diet. Dietary choices play a pivotal role in the prevention of ulcer development, as well as in supporting the healing process for those already affected.

Seniors often face unique challenges when it comes to dietary needs. This chapter explores the significance of tailoring a diet specifically for seniors dealing with stomach ulcers, taking into account factors such as nutritional requirements, digestion, and overall well-being.

The role of a specialized diet extends beyond symptom management; it contributes to the overall health and quality of life for seniors. By focusing on the nutritional aspects of care, this book aims to empower seniors to make informed and health-conscious dietary choices.

Chapter 1: Stomach Ulcers in Seniors

Overview of Stomach Ulcers

Stomach ulcers, also known as peptic ulcers, are open sores that develop on the inner lining of the stomach. These ulcers can also occur in the upper part of the small intestine and are collectively referred to as peptic ulcers. Stomach ulcers are a common medical condition that can cause various symptoms and complications if left untreated. Understanding the causes, symptoms, diagnosis, and treatment options is crucial for managing and preventing the development of stomach ulcers.

Causes of Stomach Ulcers

The most common cause of stomach ulcers is infection with the bacterium Helicobacter pylori (H. pylori). This bacterium is estimated to be present in the stomach lining of about two-thirds of the world's population. H. pylori can weaken the protective mucous layer that lines the stomach and small intestine, making it more susceptible to the corrosive effects of stomach acids.

In addition to H. pylori infection, the prolonged use of nonsteroidal anti-inflammatory drugs (NSAIDs) is another common cause of stomach ulcers. Medications such as aspirin, ibuprofen, and naproxen can irritate the stomach lining and contribute to the formation of ulcers, especially when taken over an extended period or in high doses.

While H. pylori infection and NSAID use are the primary culprits, other factors such as excessive alcohol consumption, smoking, and certain medical conditions may also increase the risk of developing stomach ulcers. Understanding and addressing these underlying causes is important for effective prevention and management of stomach ulcers.

Symptoms of Stomach Ulcers

Stomach ulcers can manifest with a variety of symptoms, and their severity can vary among individuals. Common symptoms of stomach ulcers include:

1. Burning Pain: A burning sensation or pain in the abdomen, often located between the chest and the navel, is a hallmark symptom. This pain can range from mild to severe and may occur on an empty stomach or a few hours after eating.

2. Nausea and Vomiting: Individuals with stomach ulcers may experience nausea, and in some cases, vomiting. Vomiting may contain blood or have a coffee-ground appearance if the ulcer is bleeding.

3. Indigestion: Persistent indigestion or discomfort after meals can be a symptom of stomach ulcers. This may include bloating, belching, or a feeling of fullness.

4. Loss of Appetite and Weight Loss: Stomach ulcers can lead to a decreased appetite, and over time, individuals may experience weight loss.

5. Dark Stools: Bleeding from stomach ulcers can result in black, tarry stools due to the presence of digested blood. This is known as melena.

6. Anemia: Chronic bleeding from stomach ulcers can lead to iron deficiency anemia, characterized by fatigue, weakness, and pale skin.

Diagnosis of Stomach Ulcers

1. Medical History and Physical Examination: Healthcare providers often begin by obtaining a thorough medical history and conducting a physical examination to assess symptoms and risk factors.

2. Endoscopy: A key diagnostic procedure involves using an endoscope, a flexible tube with a camera, to examine the interior of the stomach and duodenum. This allows direct visualization of ulcers and the collection of tissue samples for biopsy.

3. Upper GI Series: This imaging test involves drinking a contrast solution that helps create X-ray images of the upper gastrointestinal (GI) tract, including the stomach and duodenum.

4. Blood Tests: Blood tests may be conducted to check for the presence of H. pylori infection or to assess for signs of anemia related to bleeding ulcers.

5. Stool Tests: Stool tests may be performed to detect the presence of blood, helping to confirm or rule out gastrointestinal bleeding.

Chapter 2: The Senior's Guide to a Healing Diet

Stomach ulcers can significantly impact dietary choices, especially for seniors seeking to manage their health effectively. This chapter explores the fundamentals of a stomach ulcer-friendly diet, highlighting nutritional requirements for seniors and the importance of balancing macro and micronutrients.

Basics of a Stomach Ulcer-Friendly Diet

1. Low-Acidity Foods: Opt for foods that are low in acidity to minimize irritation to the stomach lining. This includes lean proteins, non-citrus fruits, and vegetables such as broccoli, carrots, and leafy greens.

2. High-Fiber Choices: Incorporate high-fiber foods to promote digestive health. Whole grains, legumes, and fruits like apples and berries are excellent sources of fiber that can aid in maintaining regular bowel movements.

3. Lean Proteins: Choose lean protein sources such as poultry, fish, tofu, and eggs. These proteins are easier on the digestive system and provide essential amino acids for overall health.

4. Probiotic-Rich Foods: Integrate probiotic-rich foods like yogurt, kefir, and sauerkraut to support a healthy balance of gut bacteria. Probiotics can contribute to improved digestion and strengthen the immune system.

5. Moderate Fat Intake: Opt for moderate amounts of healthy fats, such as those found in avocados, olive oil, and nuts. Avoid excessive consumption of fried and fatty foods, which can increase stomach acid production.

6. Avoid Trigger Foods: Identify and steer clear of foods that may trigger ulcer symptoms, such as spicy foods, caffeine, alcohol, and acidic beverages.

7. Small, Frequent Meals: Instead of three large meals, consider consuming smaller, more frequent meals throughout the day. This approach can help prevent excess stomach acid production and promote better digestion.

Nutritional Requirements for Seniors

1. Adequate Protein Intake: Seniors should ensure they receive sufficient protein to maintain muscle mass and overall health. This is particularly important for individuals recovering from the effects of stomach ulcers.

2. Calcium and Vitamin D: Support bone health by including calcium-rich foods (e.g., dairy, leafy greens) and ensuring adequate vitamin D intake. Vitamin D aids in calcium absorption.

3. B Vitamins: Consume foods rich in B vitamins, such as whole grains, legumes, and leafy greens, to support energy metabolism and overall well-being.

4. Hydration: Stay well-hydrated, as water is essential for digestion and helps prevent constipation, a common issue for seniors.

Balancing Macro and Micronutrients

1. **Proper** **Carbohydrate Distribution:** Choose complex carbohydrates like whole grains and vegetables, distributing them evenly throughout meals for sustained energy and stable blood sugar levels.

2. Modest Salt Use: Limit sodium intake to support heart health and prevent water retention. Utilize herbs and spices for flavor in place of too much salt.

3. Portion Control: Practice portion control to avoid overeating, which can put additional strain on the digestive system.

Chapter 3: Foods to Include

Alkaline Diet Benefits

Understanding the alkaline diet is crucial for seniors seeking to manage stomach ulcers effectively. The alkaline diet emphasizes the consumption of foods that help maintain the body's optimal pH levels, potentially alleviating symptoms associated with stomach ulcers. By creating an alkaline environment, this diet may support overall well-being and stomach health.

Alkaline-rich Foods for Seniors

To embrace the alkaline diet, seniors can incorporate a variety of alkaline-rich foods into their daily meals. Here's a comprehensive guide:

1. **Fruits:** Include alkaline fruits such as bananas, melons, and berries, which not only taste delicious but also contribute to maintaining a balanced pH.

2. **Vegetables**: Incorporate alkaline vegetables like spinach, kale, broccoli, and cucumbers. These provide essential nutrients while supporting the alkaline balance in the body.

3. **Legumes:** Opt for alkaline legumes like lentils and chickpeas, which offer a good source of protein without contributing to acidity.

4. **Nuts and Seeds**: Almonds and chia seeds are examples of alkaline-rich foods that can be added to snacks or meals for a nutrient boost.

5. **Herbs and Spices:** Choose alkaline herbs and spices like basil, thyme, and turmeric to add flavor to dishes without compromising stomach health.

Role of Anti-Inflammatory Diet in Stomach Ulcer Management

Adopting an anti-inflammatory diet is significant for managing stomach ulcers. Chronic inflammation can exacerbate symptoms, and specific dietary choices can help mitigate inflammation, reduce discomfort, and contribute to the healing process.

Anti-Inflammatory food list for seniors Foods

Seniors can build an anti-inflammatory diet by including the following foods:

1. Fatty Fish: Omega-3 fatty acids found in fish like salmon and mackerel possess anti-inflammatory properties, aiding in ulcer management.

2. Colorful Fruits and Vegetables: Berries, cherries, and leafy greens are rich in antioxidants, helping to combat inflammation and promote gastrointestinal health.

3. Whole Grains: Opt for whole grains like brown rice, quinoa, and oats, providing fiber and nutrients without causing inflammation.

4. Healthy Fats: Olive oil, avocados, and nuts contain monounsaturated fats that can help reduce inflammation and support digestive well-being.

Importance of Probiotics for Digestive Health

Probiotics play a crucial role in maintaining optimal digestive health, especially for seniors managing stomach ulcers. These beneficial bacteria contribute to a balanced gut microbiome, enhance nutrient absorption, and support the body's immune system.

Probiotic Foods Suitable for Seniors with stomach ulcer

Seniors can introduce the following probiotic-rich foods into their diet:

1. Yogurt: Choose plain, unsweetened yogurt with live cultures to promote the growth of beneficial bacteria in the gut.

2. Kefir: A fermented dairy product that provides a rich source of probiotics, supporting digestive health.

3. Kimchi: A traditional Korean dish made of fermented vegetables, including cabbage and radishes, offering a flavorful way to incorporate probiotics.

4. Fermented Vegetables: Include sauerkraut and pickles, as these fermented vegetables contain probiotics that can aid in ulcer management.

Chapter 4: Foods to Avoid

Trigger Foods for Stomach Ulcers

Stomach ulcers demand careful dietary choices, and recognizing trigger foods is essential for effective management. This section outlines common trigger foods that can exacerbate ulcer symptoms, including:

1. Spicy Foods: Explore the link between spicy foods and increased stomach acid production. Understand why individuals with stomach ulcers may experience heightened discomfort after consuming spicy dishes and the importance of limiting or avoiding them.

2. Acidic Foods and Beverages: Learn about the impact of acidic foods and beverages on the stomach lining. Citrus fruits, tomatoes, and acidic drinks can irritate ulcers, potentially leading to increased pain and inflammation.

3. Caffeine and Coffee: Explore the role of caffeine in stimulating stomach acid production and its potential to worsen ulcer symptoms. Consider alternatives to traditional coffee that may be gentler on the digestive system.

4. Alcohol: Understand the effects of alcohol on the stomach lining and how it can contribute to the development and exacerbation of stomach ulcers. This section provides insights into the importance of moderating or eliminating alcohol consumption.

5. Fried and Fatty Foods: Delve into the impact of fried and fatty foods on digestion and stomach health. Discover why these foods can be challenging for individuals with stomach ulcers and the benefits of opting for healthier cooking methods.

Understanding Acidic and Spicy Foods

Gain a comprehensive understanding of the relationship between acidic and spicy foods and stomach ulcers. This section explores the mechanisms by which these foods can aggravate ulcer symptoms, including:

1. Increased Acid Production: Examine how spicy foods and certain acidic items can stimulate the production of stomach acid, potentially leading to heightened discomfort and pain for individuals with stomach ulcers.

2. Irritation of the Stomach Lining: Understand how the consumption of acidic and spicy foods can irritate the already compromised stomach lining, contributing to inflammation and delaying the healing process.

3. Potential for Triggering Ulcer Flare-ups: Explore the role of these foods in triggering flare-ups of ulcer symptoms, hindering the progress of healing and complicating the management of stomach ulcers.

Chapter 5: Senior-Friendly Breakfast Recipes

Here are 10 delicious, nutrient-rich, and easy-to-prepare breakfast recipes designed for seniors managing stomach ulcers:

1. Banana Almond Smoothie Bowl

Ingredients
- 1 ripe banana
- 1/4 cup almonds
- 1 cup Greek yogurt (low-fat)
- 1 tablespoon honey
- 1/2 cup granola (low-sugar)

Preparation
1. Blend banana, almonds, Greek yogurt, and honey until smooth.
2. Pour into a bowl and top with granola.
3. Serves: 1
4. Nutritional Value (approx.):
   - Calories: 400
   - Protein: 20g
   - Fiber: 6g

- Healthy Fats: 15g
- Sugars: 18g

2. Oatmeal with Berries and Chia Seeds

Ingredients
- 1/2 cup rolled oats
- 1 cup almond milk
- 1/2 cup mixed berries (blueberries, strawberries)
- 1 tablespoon chia seeds
- 1 tablespoon maple syrup

Preparation
1. Cook oats in the almond milk till it turns to cream.
2. Top with mixed berries, chia seeds, and maple syrup.
3. Serves: 1
4. Nutritional Value (approx.):
   - Calories: 350
   - Protein: 10g
   - Fiber: 8g
   - Healthy Fats: 7g
   - Sugars: 12g

3. Avocado and Salmon Toast

Ingredients

- 1 slice whole-grain bread
- 1/2 avocado, mashed
- 2 oz smoked salmon
- 1 teaspoon lemon juice
- Fresh dill for garnish

Preparation

1. Toast the bread.
2. Spread mashed avocado on the toast.
3. Top with smoked salmon, drizzle with lemon juice, and garnish with fresh dill.
4. Serves: 1
5. Nutritional Value (approx.):
   - Calories: 300
   - Protein: 15g
   - Fiber: 6g
   - Healthy Fats: 15g
   - Sugars: 2g

4. Quinoa Breakfast Bowl

Ingredients

- 1/2 cup cooked quinoa
- 1/4 cup sliced almonds
- 1/2 cup mixed fresh fruit (kiwi, pineapple, mango)
- 1 tablespoon honey

Preparation

1. Combine quinoa, sliced almonds, and mixed fruit in a bowl.
2. Drizzle with honey.
3. Serves: 1
4. Nutritional Value (approx.):
   - Calories: 350
   - Protein: 8g
   - Fiber: 6g
   - Healthy Fats: 10g
   - Sugars: 20g

5. Greek Yogurt Parfait

Ingredients

- 1 cup Greek yogurt (low-fat)
- 1/2 cup granola (low-sugar)
- 1/2 cup mixed berries (raspberries, blackberries)
- 1 tablespoon honey

Preparation

1. Layer Greek yogurt, granola, and mixed berries in a glass.
2. Drizzle with honey.
3. Serves: 1
4. Nutritional Value (approx.):
   - Calories: 300
   - Protein: 20g
   - Fiber: 5g
   - Healthy Fats: 7g
   - Sugars: 15g

6. Spinach and Feta Omelette

Ingredients

- 2 large eggs
- 1/2 cup fresh spinach, chopped
- 2 tablespoons feta cheese, crumbled
- 1 teaspoon olive oil

Preparation

1. Whisk eggs and fold in spinach and feta.
2. Cook in olive oil until set.
3. Serves: 1
4. Nutritional Value (approx.):
   - Calories: 250
   - Protein: 15g
   - Fiber: 2g
   - Healthy Fats: 18g
   - Sugars: 1g

7. Blueberry Chia Seed Pudding

Ingredients

- 2 tablespoons chia seeds
- 1/2 cup almond milk
- 1/4 cup blueberries (fresh or frozen)
- 1 teaspoon vanilla extract
- 1 teaspoon maple syrup

Preparation

1. Mix chia seeds, almond milk, blueberries, vanilla extract, and maple syrup in a jar.
2. Refrigerate overnight.
3. Serves: 1
4. Nutritional Value (approx.):
   - Calories: 220
   - Protein: 6g
   - Fiber: 10g
   - Healthy Fats: 8g
   - Sugars: 8g

8. Apple Cinnamon Baked Oatmeal

Ingredients

- 1/2 cup rolled oats
- 1/2 cup almond milk
- 1/2 apple, diced
- 1 teaspoon cinnamon
- 1 tablespoon chopped walnuts

Preparation

1. Mix oats, almond milk, diced apple, and cinnamon.
2. Bake until set, and top with chopped walnuts.
3. Serves: 1
4. Nutritional Value (approx.):
   - Calories: 280
   - Protein: 7g
   - Fiber: 7g
   - Healthy Fats: 10g
   - Sugars: 10g

9. Cottage Cheese and Pineapple Bowl

Ingredients

- 1/2 cup cottage cheese
- 1/2 cup pineapple chunks
- 1 tablespoon sunflower seeds
- 1 teaspoon honey

Preparation

1. Combine cottage cheese, pineapple chunks, and sunflower seeds in a bowl.
2. Drizzle with honey.
3. Serves: 1
4. Nutritional Value (approx.):
   - Calories: 220
   - Protein: 15g
   - Fiber: 2g
   - Healthy Fats: 7g
   - Sugars: 15g

10. Sweet Potato and Turkey Hash

Ingredients

- 1/2 cup sweet potato, grated
- 3 oz ground turkey
- 1/4 cup bell peppers, diced
- 1 teaspoon olive oil
- 1/2 teaspoon paprika

Preparation

1. Cook sweet potato, ground turkey, and bell peppers in olive oil until cooked through.
2. Sprinkle it with paprika.
3. Serves: 1
4. Nutritional Value (approx.):
   - Calories: 320
   - Protein: 18g
   - Fiber: 5g
   - Healthy Fats: 10g
   - Sugars: 5g

Chapter 6: Senior-Friendly Lunch Recipes

Here are 10 delicious, nutrient-rich, and easy-to-prepare lunch recipes designed for seniors managing stomach ulcers:

1. Grilled Salmon with Quinoa Salad

Ingredients

- 4 oz salmon filet
- 1/2 cup quinoa, cooked
- 1 cup mixed greens (spinach, arugula)
- 1/4 cup cherry tomatoes, halved
- 1 tablespoon olive oil
- Lemon wedges for garnish

Preparation

1. Grill the salmon until cooked.
2. Mix cooked quinoa, mixed greens, cherry tomatoes, and olive oil.
3. Serve the grilled salmon on top of the quinoa salad, garnish with lemon wedges.
4. Serves: 1
5. Nutritional Value (approx.):

- Calories: 400
- Protein: 25g
- Fiber: 5g
- Healthy Fats: 15g
- Sugars: 2g

2. Turkey and Avocado Wrap

Ingredients

- 4 oz turkey breast slices
- 1 whole-grain wrap
- 1/2 avocado, sliced
- 1/4 cup cucumber, thinly sliced
- 1 tablespoon Greek yogurt
- Lettuce leaves for wrapping

Preparation

1. Layer turkey, avocado, cucumber, and Greek yogurt on the wrap.
2. Roll the ingredients in a lettuce leaf or whole-grain wrap.
3. Serves: 1
4. Nutritional Value (approx.):
   - Calories: 350
   - Protein: 20g
   - Fiber: 8g
   - Healthy Fats: 15g

- Sugars: 3g

3. Quinoa and Vegetable Stir-Fry

Ingredients

- 1/2 cup quinoa, cooked
- 1 cup mixed vegetables (bell peppers, broccoli, carrots)
- 3 oz tofu, cubed
- 1 tablespoon soy sauce
- 1 teaspoon sesame oil

Preparation

1. Stir-fry mixed vegetables and tofu in sesame oil.
2. Add cooked quinoa and soy sauce, stir until well combined.
3. Serves: 1
4. Nutritional Value (approx.):
   - Calories: 350
   - Protein: 15g
   - Fiber: 8g
   - Healthy Fats: 10g
   - Sugars: 5g

4. Spinach and Chickpea Salad

Ingredients

- 2 cups fresh spinach
- 1/2 cup chickpeas, cooked
- 1/4 cup feta cheese, crumbled
- 1/4 cup cherry tomatoes, halved
- 1 tablespoon balsamic vinaigrette

Preparation

1. Toss fresh spinach, chickpeas, feta cheese, and cherry tomatoes.
2. Drizzle with balsamic vinaigrette.
3. Serves: 1
4. Nutritional Value (approx.):
   - Calories: 300
   - Protein: 12g
   - Fiber: 8g
   - Healthy Fats: 10g
   - Sugars: 4g

5. Lentil Soup with Whole-Grain Bread

Ingredients
- 1 cup lentils, cooked
- 1/2 cup carrots, diced
- 1/2 cup celery, diced
- 1/2 cup onions, chopped
- 2 cups low-sodium vegetable broth
- Whole-grain bread for serving

Preparation
1. Cook lentils, carrots, celery, and onions in vegetable broth until vegetables are tender.
2. Serves: 1
3. Nutritional Value (approx.):
    - Calories: 320
    - Protein: 18g
    - Fiber: 14g
    - Healthy Fats: 3g
    - Sugars: 4g

6. Chicken and Vegetable Skewers with Quinoa

Ingredients

- 4 oz chicken breast, cubed
- 1/2 cup bell peppers, cut into chunks
- 1/2 cup zucchini, sliced
- 1/2 cup cherry tomatoes
- 1/2 cup quinoa, cooked
- 1 tablespoon olive oil

Preparation

1. Thread chicken, bell peppers, zucchini, and cherry tomatoes onto skewers.

2. Grill until chicken is cooked.

3. Serve over cooked quinoa, drizzle with olive oil.

4. Serves: 1

5. Nutritional Value (approx.):
   - Calories: 380
   - Protein: 25g
   - Fiber: 6g
   - Healthy Fats: 12g
   - Sugars: 4g

7. Shrimp and Broccoli Stir-Fry

Ingredients

- 4 oz shrimp, peeled and deveined
- 1 cup broccoli florets

- 1/2 cup brown rice, cooked
- 1 tablespoon low-sodium soy sauce
- 1 teaspoon sesame oil

Preparation

1. Stir-fry shrimp and broccoli in sesame oil.
2. Add cooked brown rice and soy sauce, stir until well combined.
3. Serves: 1
4. Nutritional Value (approx.):
   - Calories: 320
   - Protein: 20g
   - Fiber: 6g
   - Healthy Fats: 8g
   - Sugars: 2g

8. Greek Salad with Grilled Chicken

Ingredients

- 4 oz grilled chicken breast, sliced
- 2 cups mixed greens (romaine, cucumber, olives)
- 1/4 cup feta cheese, crumbled
- 1/4 cup cherry tomatoes, halved
- 1 tablespoon olive oil
- Lemon wedges for garnish

Preparation

1. Toss mixed greens, feta cheese, and cherry tomatoes.
2. Top with grilled chicken slices, drizzle with olive oil, and garnish with lemon wedges.
3. Serves: 1
4. Nutritional Value (approx.):
   - Calories: 350
   - Protein: 25g
   - Fiber: 6g
   - Healthy Fats: 15g
   - Sugars: 3g

9. Vegetable and Tofu Stir-Fry with Brown Rice

Ingredients

- 1 cup of mixed vegetables (snap peas, broccoli, bell peppers,)
- 3 oz tofu, cubed
- 1/2 cup brown rice, cooked
- 1 tablespoon low-sodium soy sauce
- 1 teaspoon ginger, minced

Preparation

1. Stir-fry mixed vegetables and tofu in soy sauce and ginger.
2. Serve over cooked brown rice.
3. Serves: 1
4. Nutritional Value (approx.):
   - Calories: 320
   - Protein: 15g
   - Fiber: 8g
   - Healthy Fats: 10g
   - Sugars: 4g

10. Egg and Vegetable Wrap

Ingredients

- 2 large eggs, scrambled
- 1 whole-grain wrap
- 1/4 cup bell peppers, diced
- 1/4 cup tomatoes, diced
- 1 tablespoon feta cheese, crumbled
- 1 teaspoon olive oil

Preparation

1. Scramble eggs and cook in olive oil.
2. Fill the wrap with scrambled eggs, bell peppers, tomatoes, and feta cheese.
3. Serves: 1
4. Nutritional Value (approx.):
   - Calories: 300
   - Protein: 18g
   - Fiber: 5g
   - Healthy Fats: 12g
   - Sugars: 3g

1. Baked Salmon and Steamed Vegetables with Quinoa

Ingredients

4 salmon filets

1 cup quinoa

2 cups mixed vegetables (carrots, zucchini, broccoli)

Olive oil, lemon juice, salt, and pepper for seasoning

Preparation

Preheat the oven to 375°F (190°C).

Season salmon with olive oil, lemon juice, salt, and pepper. Bake for 15-20 minutes.

Cook quinoa according to package instructions.

Steam mixed vegetables.

Serve salmon over a bed of quinoa with steamed vegetables on the side.

Servings: 4

Nutritional Value: High in omega-3 fatty acids, protein, fiber, vitamins, and minerals.
Cooking Time: 30 minutes.

2. Ginger-Turmeric Chicken Stir-Fry

Ingredients
1 lb chicken breast, thinly sliced
2 cups broccoli florets
1 bell pepper, thinly sliced
2 tsp grated ginger
1 tsp turmeric powder
Low-sodium soy sauce
Preparation
Stir-fry chicken until cooked. Set aside.
In the same pan, stir-fry vegetables with ginger and turmeric.
Add cooked chicken back to the pan. Season with soy sauce.
Stir until well combined and heated through.
Servings: 4
Nutritional Value: Anti-inflammatory properties from ginger and turmeric, lean protein, vitamins, and fiber.

Cooking Time: 20 minutes.

3. Mango and Spinach Salad with Grilled Chicken

Ingredients

2 cups baby spinach

1 ripe mango, sliced

1 grilled chicken breast, sliced

1/4 cup walnuts

Olive oil and balsamic vinegar for dressing

Preparation

Toss baby spinach, mango slices, grilled chicken, and walnuts in a bowl.

Sprinkle it with a mixture of balsamic vinegar and olive oil.

Servings: 2

Nutritional Value: Rich in antioxidants, vitamin C, fiber, and lean protein.

Cooking Time: 15 minutes.

4. Turkey and Vegetable Skewers with Quinoa

Ingredients

1 lb turkey breast, cut into cubes

Cherry tomatoes, bell peppers, and red onions for skewers

1 cup quinoa

Olive oil, lemon juice, salt, and pepper for marinade

Preparation

Marinate turkey cubes in olive oil, lemon juice, salt, and pepper. Skewer with vegetables.

Grill until the turkey is cooked.

Cook quinoa according to package instructions.

Servings: 4

Nutritional Value: Lean protein, fiber, vitamins, and minerals.

Cooking Time: 25 minutes.

5. Sweet Potato and Carrot Soup

Ingredients

2 sweet potatoes, peeled and diced

2 carrots, peeled and sliced

1 onion, chopped

1 clove garlic, minced

Vegetable broth, salt, and pepper

Preparation

Sauté onions and garlic until soft.

Add sweet potatoes and carrots. Cook for 5 minutes.

Pour in enough vegetable broth to cover vegetables. Simmer until the veggies are tender.

Blend until smooth. Season with salt and pepper.

Servings: 4

Nutritional Value: Rich in beta-carotene, fiber, and antioxidants.

Cooking Time: 30 minutes.

6. Ginger Chicken Rice Bowl

Ingredients

1 cup cooked brown rice

1 cup shredded cooked chicken breast

1 tablespoon grated fresh ginger

1 cup steamed broccoli

1 tablespoon low-sodium soy sauce

1 teaspoon sesame oil

Preparation

Combine cooked rice, shredded chicken, ginger, steamed broccoli, soy sauce, and sesame oil in a bowl. Mix well.

Servings: 2

Nutritional Value (per serving):

Calories: 350

Protein: 25g

Fiber: 4g

Vitamin C: 90mg

Cooking Time: 20 minutes

7. Quinoa and Vegetable Stir-Fry

Ingredients

1 cup cooked quinoa

1 cup mixed stir-fry vegetables (bell peppers, zucchini, carrots)

1 tablespoon olive oil

2 cloves minced garlic

1 teaspoon turmeric

Salt and pepper to taste

Preparation

Sauté garlic in olive oil, add mixed vegetables, cooked quinoa, turmeric, salt, and pepper. Stir-fry until vegetables are tender.

Servings: 2

Nutritional Value (per serving):

Calories: 300

Protein: 10g

Fiber: 8g

Vitamin A: 1500IU

Cooking Time: 15 minutes

8. Baked Salmon with Sweet Potato Mash

Ingredients
2 salmon filets
2 medium sweet potatoes, peeled and cubed
1 tablespoon olive oil
1 teaspoon rosemary
Lemon wedges for serving
Preparation
Bake salmon with rosemary at 375°F (190°C) for 15-20 minutes. Boil sweet potatoes until tender, mash with olive oil.
Servings: 2
Nutritional Value (per serving):
Calories: 400
Protein: 30g
Omega-3 Fatty Acids: 1.5g
Cooking Time: 25 minutes

9. Spinach and Feta Stuffed Chicken Breast

Ingredients

2 boneless, skinless chicken breasts
1 cup fresh spinach
2 tablespoons crumbled feta cheese
1 teaspoon oregano
Salt and pepper to taste

Preparation

Make a pocket in each chicken breast, stuff with spinach, feta, oregano, salt, and pepper. Bake at high temperature up to 190°C for at least 25-30 minutes.

Servings: 2
Nutritional Value (per serving):
Calories: 280
Protein: 35g
Calcium: 200mg
Cooking Time: 30 minutes

10. Lentil and Vegetable Soup

Ingredients

1 cup dried green lentils, rinsed

1 onion, diced

2 carrots, sliced

2 celery stalks, chopped

1 teaspoon cumin

1 teaspoon turmeric

4 cups vegetable broth

Preparation

Combine all ingredients in a pot, bring to a boil, then simmer until lentils are tender.

Servings: 4

Nutritional Value (per serving):

Calories: 290

Protein: 35g

Calcium: 200mg

Cooking Time: 25 minutes

Chapter 8: Senior-Friendly snacks Recipes

These snack recipes include ingredients that are generally considered gentle on the stomach, but individual tolerances may vary.

1. Banana and Almond Butter Toast

Ingredients
- 1 slice whole-grain bread
- 1 ripe banana, sliced
- 1 tablespoon almond butter

Preparation
Toast the bread with toaster, spread it with almond butter, and top it with banana cuts.
Servings: 1
Nutritional Value (per serving):
Calories: 250
Fiber: 5g
Potassium: 450mg
Preparation Time: 5 minutes

2. Greek Yogurt with Honey and Walnuts

Ingredients
- 1 cup plain Greek yogurt
- 1 tablespoon honey
- 2 tablespoons chopped walnuts

Preparation
Top Greek yogurt with honey and chopped walnuts.
Servings: 1
Nutritional Value (per serving):
Calories: 200
Protein: 20g
Calcium: 200mg
Preparation Time: 2 minutes

3. Apple Slices with Cottage Cheese

Ingredients
- 1 medium apple, sliced
- 1/2 cup low-fat cottage cheese

Preparation
Serve apple slices with a side of cottage cheese.
Servings: 1

Nutritional Value (per serving):
Calories: 150
Protein: 10g
Vitamin C: 8mg
Preparation Time: 5 minutes

4. Steamed Edamame with Sea Salt

Ingredients
- 1 cup edamame (soybeans), steamed
- Sea salt to taste
Preparation
Gently heat edamame and drizzle it with sea salt.
Servings: 1
Nutritional Value (per serving):
Calories: 120
Protein: 11g
Fiber: 8g
Preparation Time: 5 minutes

5. Rice Cake with Avocado and Tomato

Ingredients
- 1 rice cake
- 1/2 ripe avocado, mashed
- 1 small tomato, sliced

Preparation
Spread mashed avocado on the rice cake
and top with sliced tomatoes.
Servings: 1
Nutritional Value (per serving):
Calories: 180
Fiber: 5g
Vitamin K: 15mcg
Preparation Time: 5 minutes

6. Baked Sweet Potato Chips

Ingredients
- 1 sweet potato, thinly sliced
- 1 tablespoon olive oil
- Sea salt to taste

Preparation

Toss sweet potato slices in olive oil, bake at 375°F (190°C) until crispy. Sprinkle it with sea salt.

Servings: 2

Nutritional Value (per serving):

Calories: 100

Fiber: 3g

Vitamin A: 200% DV

Cooking Time: 20 minutes

7. Berry and Spinach Smoothie

Ingredients

- 1 cup fresh or frozen mixed berries
- 1 cup fresh spinach leaves
- 1/2 cup plain Greek yogurt
- 1 tablespoon honey

Preparation

Blend berries, spinach, Greek yogurt, and honey until smooth.

Servings: 1

Nutritional Value (per serving):

Calories: 150

Protein: 10g

Vitamin C: 30mg

Preparation Time: 5 minutes

8. Cucumber and Hummus Rolls

Ingredients
- 1 large cucumber, thinly sliced
- 1/4 cup hummus

Preparation
Spread hummus on cucumber slices and roll them up.
Servings: 1
Nutritional Value (per serving):
Calories: 80
Fiber: 3g
Protein: 4g
Preparation Time: 5 minutes

9. Oatmeal and Banana Muffins

Ingredients
- 1 cup rolled oats
- 2 ripe bananas, mashed
- 1/4 cup honey
- 1/2 teaspoon cinnamon

Preparation

Mix oats, mashed bananas, honey, and cinnamon. Spoon into muffin cups and bake at 350°F (175°C) for 15-20 minutes.

Servings: 6

Nutritional Value (per serving):

Calories: 120

Fiber: 2g

Potassium: 200mg

Cooking Time: 20 minutes

10. Chia Seed Pudding with Berries

Ingredients

- 2 tablespoons chia seeds
- 1/2 cup almond milk
- 1/2 teaspoon vanilla extract
- 1/2 cup mixed berries

Preparation

Mix chia seeds, almond milk, and vanilla extract. Leave in the fridge overnight. Top with mixed berries before serving.

Servings: 1

Nutritional Value (per serving):

Calories: 150

Fiber: 8g
Omega-3 Fatty Acids: 2g
Preparation Time: 5 minutes (plus chilling time)

Chapter 9: Meal Planning for Seniors

Creating Balanced Meal Plans

Meal planning for seniors is a crucial aspect of promoting overall health and well-being. As individuals age, their nutritional needs may change, and it becomes essential to focus on creating balanced meal plans that provide the necessary nutrients. Here are key considerations when developing meal plans for seniors:

1. Varied Nutrients: Aim for a variety of nutrients from different food groups, including fruits, vegetables, whole grains, lean proteins, and dairy or dairy alternatives. This helps ensure seniors receive a broad spectrum of vitamins, minerals, and essential nutrients necessary for their health.

2. Portion Control: Seniors may have different caloric needs, and portion control becomes vital to prevent overeating. Smaller, more frequent meals throughout the day can be beneficial, providing sustained energy without causing discomfort.

3. Hydration: Adequate hydration is essential for seniors, as dehydration can lead to various health issues. Include water, herbal teas, and hydrating foods like fruits and soups in the meal plan.

4. Calcium and Vitamin D: Bone health becomes increasingly important with age. Incorporate sources of calcium and vitamin D, such as dairy products, fortified foods, and leafy greens, to support bone strength.

5. Fiber-Rich Foods: Include fiber-rich foods like whole grains, legumes, fruits, and vegetables to promote digestive health. Fiber can also help manage weight and prevent constipation, which is common among seniors.

6. Healthy Fats: Choose sources of healthy fats, such as avocados, nuts, seeds, and olive oil, to support heart health. Fatty fish, flaxseed and walnuts which are the source of Omega-3 fatty acids can be particularly superior.

7. Limit Sodium and Processed Foods: Seniors should be mindful of their sodium intake to manage blood pressure. Reduce the consumption of processed and packaged foods, which often contain high levels of sodium.

8. Consider Special Dietary Needs: Some seniors may have specific dietary requirements or restrictions due to medical conditions. Consult with healthcare professionals or registered dietitians to tailor meal plans to individual needs.

Tips for Easy and Digestible Meals

Creating meals that are both easy to prepare and gentle on the digestive system is essential for seniors, especially those with stomach ulcers or digestive sensitivities. Here are practical tips for achieving this:

1. Soft and Cooked Foods: Opt for softer and well-cooked foods that are easier to chew and digest. This includes steamed vegetables, lean proteins, and whole grains that are thoroughly cooked.

2. Smaller, Frequent Meals: Rather than three large meals, consider offering smaller, more frequent meals throughout the day. This can help prevent feelings of fullness and discomfort.

3. Include Probiotics: Incorporate foods rich in probiotics, such as yogurt with live cultures or fermented foods like sauerkraut. Probiotics can support gut health and aid digestion.

4. Avoid Spicy and Acidic Foods: Limit the use of spices, spicy foods, and acidic ingredients, as these can irritate the digestive tract. Opt for milder seasonings and herbs for flavor.

5. Hydration with Meals: Encourage hydration, but avoid excessive consumption during meals, as it may interfere with digestion. Sipping water between meals is preferable.

6. Choose Lean Proteins: Opt for lean protein sources such as poultry, fish, tofu, and legumes. These are generally easier to digest compared to high-fat or heavily processed proteins.

7. Limit Gas-Producing Foods: Some foods can contribute to gas and bloating. Minimize the intake of gas-producing vegetables like cabbage and broccoli, and consider cooking them to make them more digestible.

8. Mindful Eating Practices: Encourage seniors to eat slowly, chew food thoroughly, and pay attention to hunger and fullness cues. This can help in digestion and at the same time prevents overeating.

9. Simple Cooking Techniques: Stick to simple cooking methods such as baking, steaming, or boiling, which are gentler on the digestive system compared to frying or grilling.

10. Individual Preferences and Tolerances: Consider individual preferences and tolerances when planning meals. Be open to adjusting the meal plan based on the senior's feedback and needs.

Chapter 10: Lifestyle Tips for Managing Stomach Ulcers

Stress Reduction Techniques

Effective stress management is vital for individuals dealing with stomach ulcers. Consider incorporating the following techniques:

1. Deep Breathing: Practice deep, diaphragmatic breathing to reduce stress and promote relaxation.

2. Mindfulness Meditation: Engage in mindfulness meditation to enhance awareness and manage stress levels.

3. Gentle Exercise: Include low-impact exercises like walking or yoga to alleviate stress and promote overall well-being.

4. Time Management: Organize daily tasks to minimize stressors and create a more balanced lifestyle.

Hydration and its Role

Proper hydration plays a crucial role in managing stomach ulcers. Consider these hydration tips:

1. Consistent Water Intake: Ensure regular water consumption throughout the day to maintain hydration levels.

2. Avoid Irritants: Limit or avoid caffeinated and acidic beverages, as they can irritate the stomach lining.

3. Herbal Teas: Opt for soothing herbal teas like chamomile or ginger, which may aid digestion and provide comfort.

4. Water-Rich Foods: Include water-rich foods like fruits and vegetables to contribute to overall hydration.

5. Monitor Urine Color: Check urine color; light yellow indicates proper hydration, while dark yellow may signal dehydration.

Concclusion

Our focus has been on fostering digestive wellness in seniors, particularly those managing stomach ulcers. We've explored the intricacies of crafting balanced meal plans and implementing lifestyle adjustments to enhance overall well-being.

The journey toward digestive health involves a harmonious blend of mindful nutrition, stress management, and hydration practices. By tailoring meal plans to individual needs, emphasizing nutrient-rich choices, and incorporating stress reduction techniques, caregivers and seniors can embark on a path that not only addresses stomach ulcers but also supports holistic health.

Remember, the information provided here serves as a guide, and individual responses may vary. It is crucial to consult with healthcare professionals and registered dietitians for personalized advice. By embracing a proactive approach to digestive wellness, seniors can savor a higher quality of life, enjoying meals that nourish both the body and the spirit.

May this guide serve as a compass, guiding you towards sustainable practices that promote digestive health and, ultimately, a vibrant and fulfilling senior life. Here's to a future filled with good health, wholesome meals, and the joy of savoring each moment.

www.ingramcontent.com/pod-product-compliance
Lightning Source LLC
Chambersburg PA
CBHW061010260726
48661CB00005B/2142